THE HEART

The Kids' Question and Answer Book

J. Willis Hurst, M.D. and Stuart D. Hurst

Illustrated by Patricia Wynne with Patsy Bryan and Shawna Todd

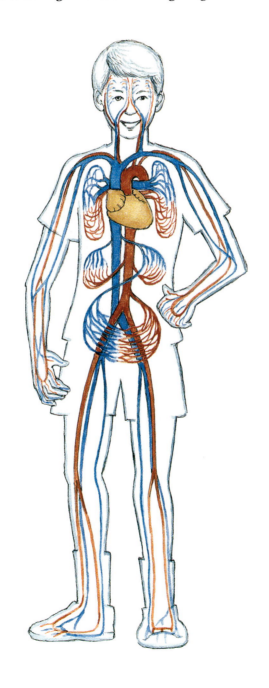

McGraw-Hill

New York   San Francisco   Washington, D.C.   Auckland   Bogotá   Caracas   Lisbon   London   Madrid
Mexico City   Milan   Montreal   New Delhi   San Juan   Singapore   Sydney   Tokyo   Toronto

This book is dedicated to kids
who want to learn about their heart
and how to protect it

McGraw-Hill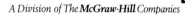

A Division of The **McGraw·Hill** *Companies*

©1999 by The McGraw-Hill Companies, Inc.

Printed in the United States of America. All rights reserved. The publisher takes no responsibility for the use of any materials or methods described in this book, nor for the products thereof.

The activities described in this book are intended for children under the direct supervision of adults. The publisher cannot be held responsible for any accidents or injuries that might result from conducting the activities without proper supervision, from not specifically following directions, or from ignoring the cautions contained in the text.

pbk 1 2 3 4 5 6 7 8 9 KGP/KGP 9 0 3 2 1 0 9 8

ISBN 0-07-031829-8

Product or brand names used in this book may be trade names or trademarks. Where we believe that there may be proprietary claims to such trade names or trademarks, the name has been used with an initial capital or it has been capitalized in the style used by the name claimant. Regardless of the capitalization used, all such names have been used in an editorial manner without any intent to convey endorsement of or other affiliation with the name claimant. Neither the author nor the publisher intends to express any judgment as to the validity or legal status of any such proprietary claims.

Printed and bound by Quebecor/Kingsport.

McGraw-Hill books are available at special quantity discounts. For more information, please write to the Director of Special Sales, McGraw-Hill, 11 West 19th Street, New York, NY 10011. Or contact your local bookstore.

Technical reviewer: Dr. Donald M. Silver
Production supervisor: Clara B. Stanley
Editing supervisor: Maureen B. Walker
Designer: Jaclyn J. Boone

PREFACE
A Family Affair

The story you are about to read is not true, but all the facts in it about your heart are true. The characters in it are not real, but they're like people who are real: my grandson, Stuart; my granddaughter, Jessica; and me. When Stuart was learning to talk he could not say grand, so he called me "Anndaddy." I'm not a camp doctor, but I am a real doctor whose specialty is the human heart. You'll see all of this in the book you are about to read.

This book began when Stuart came to visit me one day in my library when he was ten. He was full of questions, and I would frequently say, "Let's look it up." He would find the answers in a book and we would read them together. On this particular day, Stuart told me he wanted to do a science project on the heart. "What do you want to know?" I asked. Then he came up with so many questions that I said, "The answers would fill a book!"

"OK," Stuart said, "let's write a book."

So that is what we did. We wrote a book, with Stuart providing the questions and me providing the answers, rewriting until I was sure he understood. This book uses Stuart's questions as well as some from others we thought kids would like answered.

But we hope everyone, young and old, can learn something from this book. It's never too early or too late to learn to appreciate your heart. If we care for it properly, we can go a long way toward preventing heart disease, the nation's number one killer. There's no question THAT makes good sense!

I wish to thank Robert P. McGraw for his help in making this book possible. I especially want to acknowledge Jackie Ball's significant contribution to the appeal of the book through her creation of a story line and skilled simplification of sometimes complicated content. I also wish to thank Judith Terrill-Breuer of McGraw-Hill for her help in producing this book. Judith's skill, kindness, and expertise were apparent throughout the writing and publishing process. I thank Griffin Hansbury at McGraw-Hill for helping with the final push on the book. Good books are made better by good illustrations; accordingly, I thank Patricia Wynne for creating the illustrations of the children and me, and Patsy Bryan and Shawna Todd of Emory University for creating the scientific illustrations. Stuart and I could not have completed the book without the help of these experts. Finally, I wish to thank my wife Nelie, who is Stuart's "Annmommy," and Stuart's mom and dad for encouraging us to "finish the book."

J. Willis Hurst, M.D.
Emory University
Atlanta, Georgia

WHERE DOES BLOOD COME FROM?

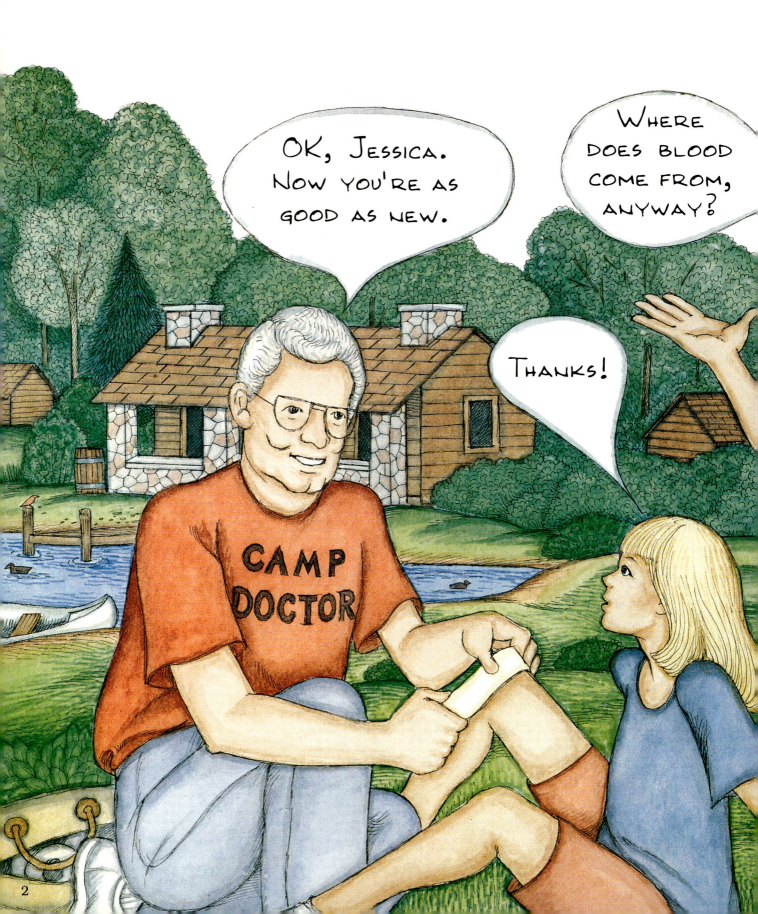

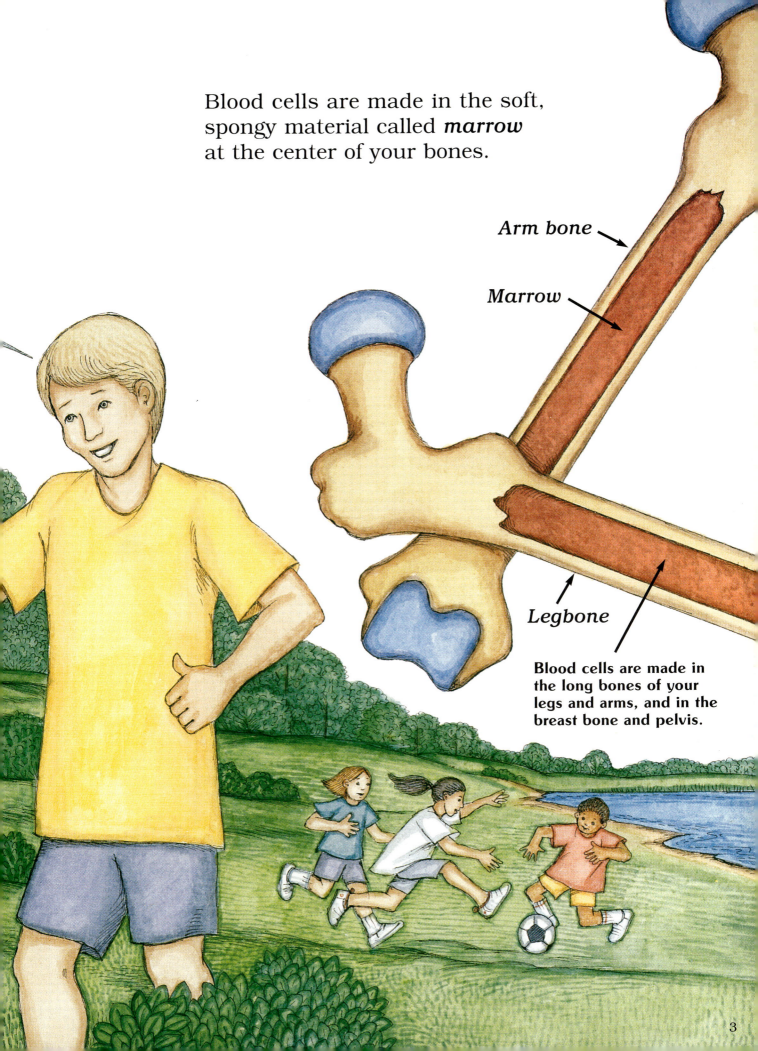

Blood cells are made in the soft, spongy material called *marrow* at the center of your bones.

Arm bone

Marrow

Legbone

Blood cells are made in the long bones of your legs and arms, and in the breast bone and pelvis.

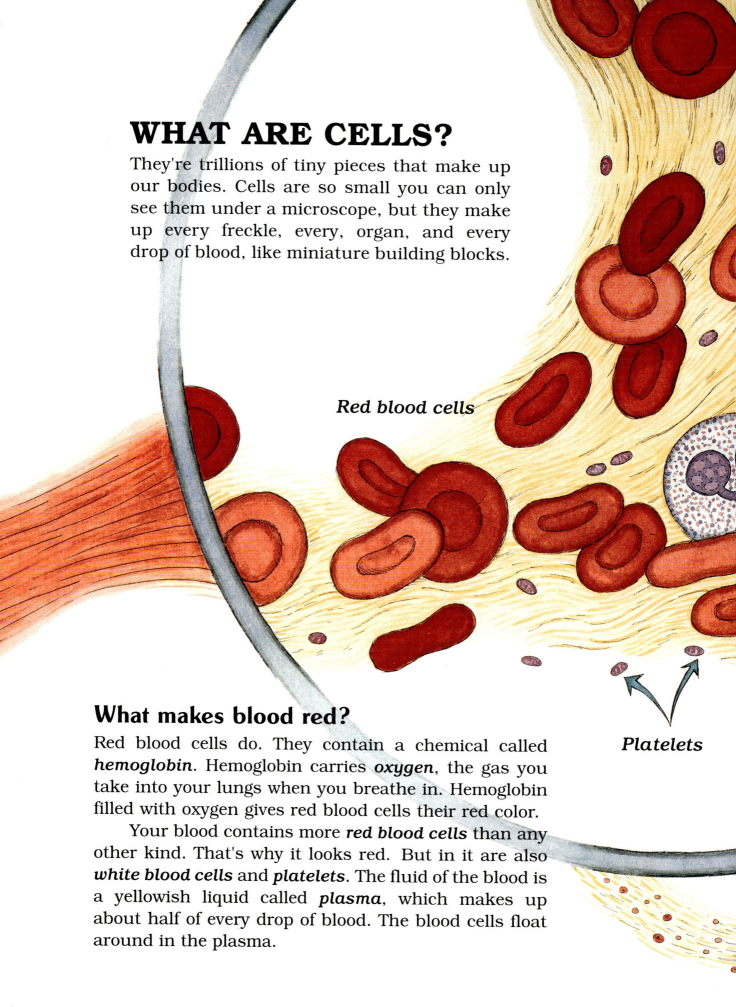

WHAT ARE CELLS?

They're trillions of tiny pieces that make up our bodies. Cells are so small you can only see them under a microscope, but they make up every freckle, every, organ, and every drop of blood, like miniature building blocks.

Red blood cells

Platelets

What makes blood red?

Red blood cells do. They contain a chemical called **hemoglobin**. Hemoglobin carries *oxygen*, the gas you take into your lungs when you breathe in. Hemoglobin filled with oxygen gives red blood cells their red color.

Your blood contains more *red blood cells* than any other kind. That's why it looks red. But in it are also *white blood cells* and *platelets*. The fluid of the blood is a yellowish liquid called *plasma*, which makes up about half of every drop of blood. The blood cells float around in the plasma.

White blood cells

Plasma

It doesn't hurt! Really!

Drop by Drop
How many red blood cells
does one drop of blood contain?

Hundreds of millions!

More! More!
Red blood cells work so hard
that they wear out
after only a few months
and need to be replaced.

Healthy bone marrow
can make millions more
in a few seconds.

Not every bone
makes blood cells!

New cells out

Leg bone

Bone marrow

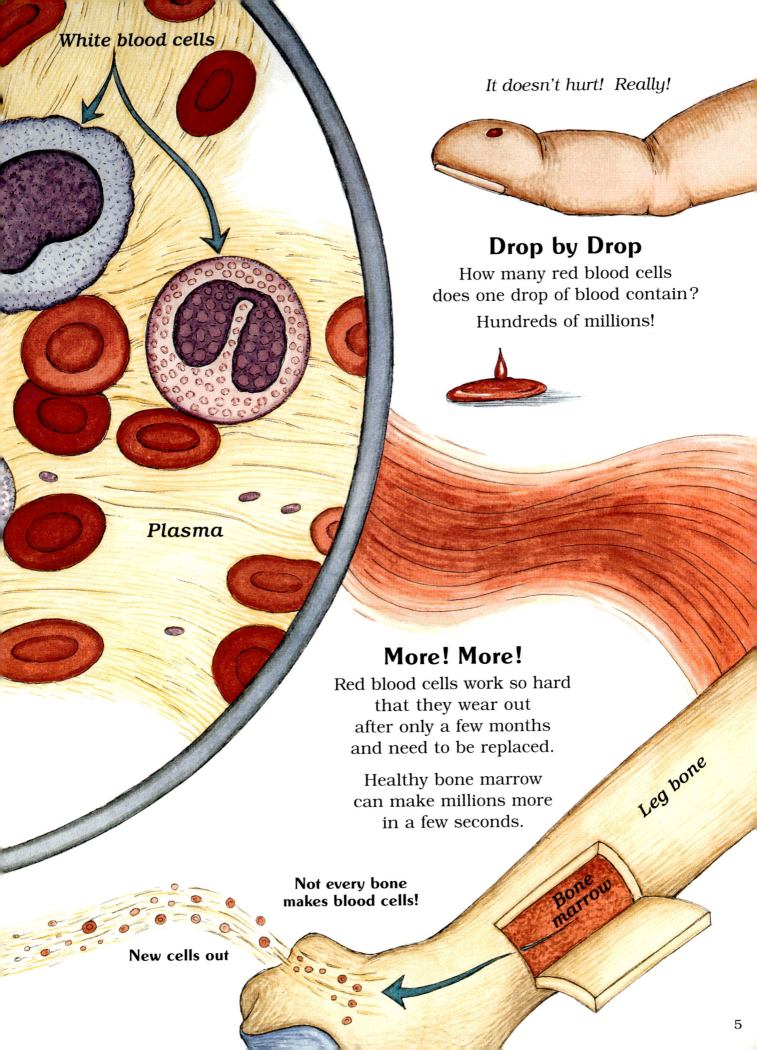

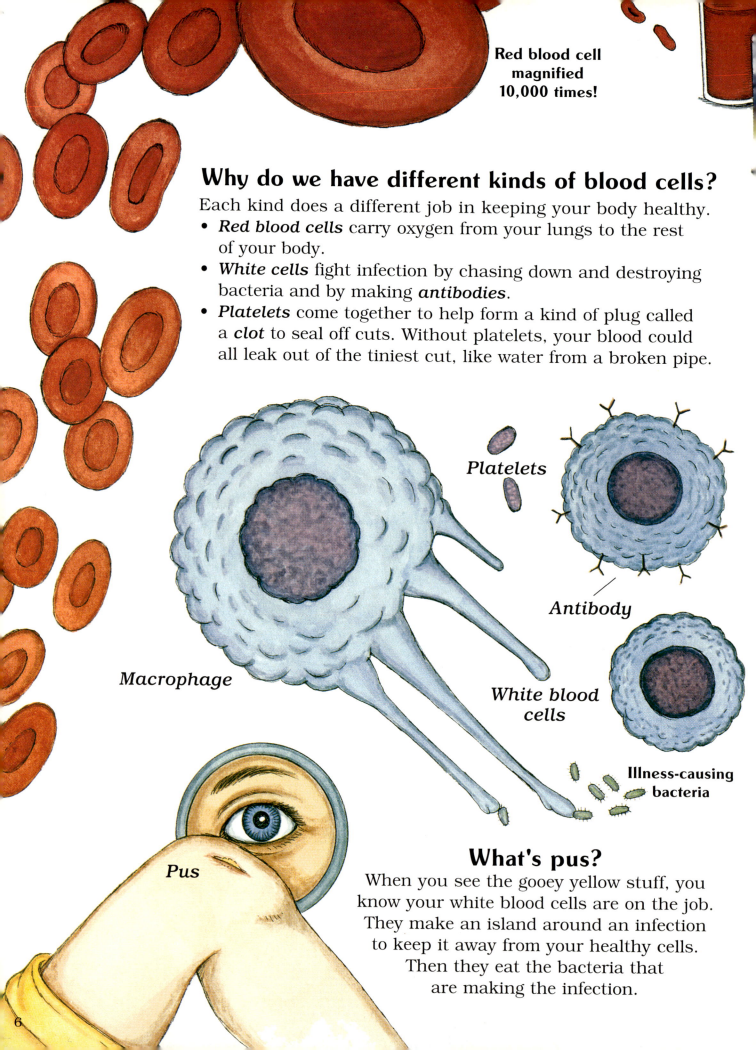

Red blood cell magnified 10,000 times!

Why do we have different kinds of blood cells?

Each kind does a different job in keeping your body healthy.

- *Red blood cells* carry oxygen from your lungs to the rest of your body.
- *White cells* fight infection by chasing down and destroying bacteria and by making *antibodies*.
- *Platelets* come together to help form a kind of plug called a *clot* to seal off cuts. Without platelets, your blood could all leak out of the tiniest cut, like water from a broken pipe.

Platelets

Antibody

Macrophage

White blood cells

Illness-causing bacteria

Pus

What's pus?

When you see the gooey yellow stuff, you know your white blood cells are on the job. They make an island around an infection to keep it away from your healthy cells. Then they eat the bacteria that are making the infection.

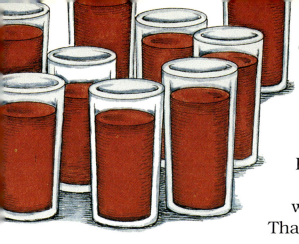

If all the blood ran out of me, how much would that be?

It depends on how much of YOU there is!
If you weighed a hundred pounds, you
would have about three and a half quarts.
That's almost enough to fill two half-gallon milk
containers or more than a dozen water glasses.

Does our blood stand still inside us?

Not for one split-second. Your blood is
constantly moving through your body.
Just press your first and second fingers on
the inside of your wrist. That throbbing is
called a *pulse*. It is caused by the action of blood
being pumped around your body by the heartbeat.

What pumps the blood?

A tireless muscle sends blood to all parts of your
body. It's totally devoted to you night and day
and never stops trying to keep you healthy. You
might say it's at the *heart* of you: your heart.

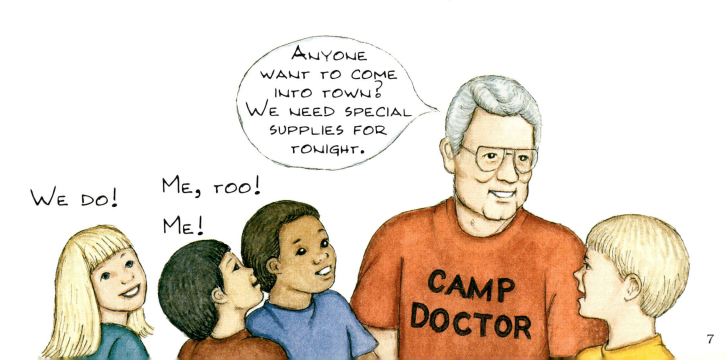

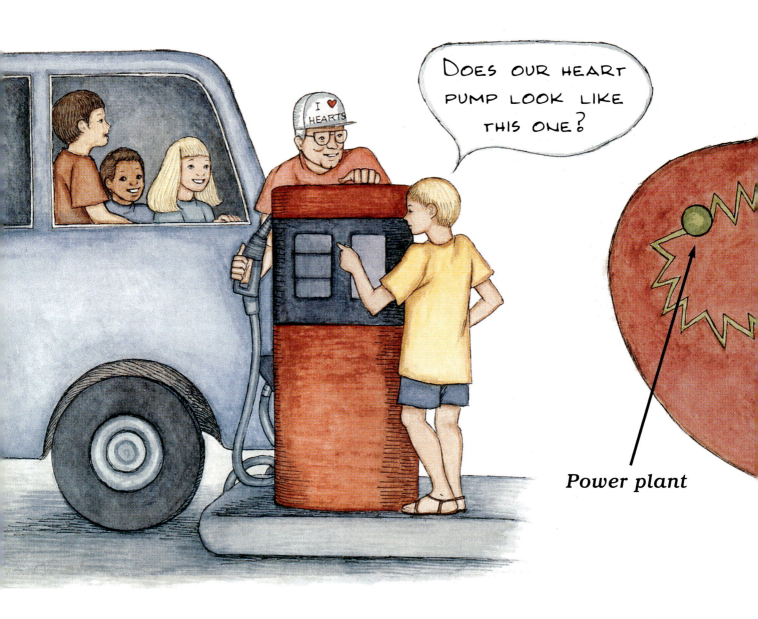

Power plant

Does our heart look like a gas pump?

No, but it serves the same purpose. We pump gas into a car's fuel tank so it can go. It's as if we were *feeding* the car with gas. Your heart pumps blood around your body, 100,000 times every day, so YOU can go. Every cell in your body needs blood to "feed" it with oxygen, proteins, and other nutrients. Without that feeding, your cells could not work. They would die.

What turns on the heart's pump? What makes it go?

The same thing that turns on your computer and keeps your frozen yogurt frozen: electricity. But people don't need to be plugged in. The heart has its own power plant called the *sinus node* that makes electricity. Seventy to eighty times a minute, there is a surge of electric power from the node that makes the heart muscle squeeze blood out into tubes called *blood vessels*. The vessels carry blood all around your body.

Is our heart really shaped like a valentine?

Your heart looks only the slightest bit like a lopsided valentine. But a better way to think of it is to imagine a two-story house — a tiny house the size of your fist.

Wait a minute! How can a heart look like a house?

Your heart doesn't *look* like a house, but it's built something like one—a tilted house with two floors and four rooms, or *chambers*. It also has two front doors.

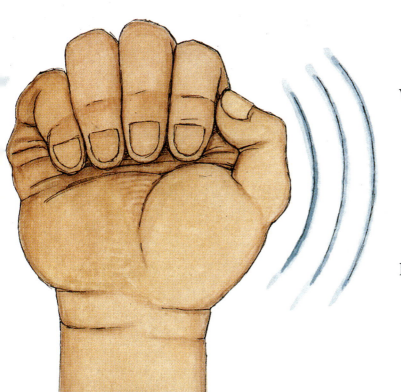

Tight squeeze

Want to know what it's like to be your heart? Make a fist. Now squeeze for one second, and relax for one second. Squeeze, relax. Squeeze, relax. Come on, keep going. Do it seventy or eighty times. Getting tired? Well, your heart has to do that EVERY MINUTE. Over your lifetime it will pump two and a half billion times.

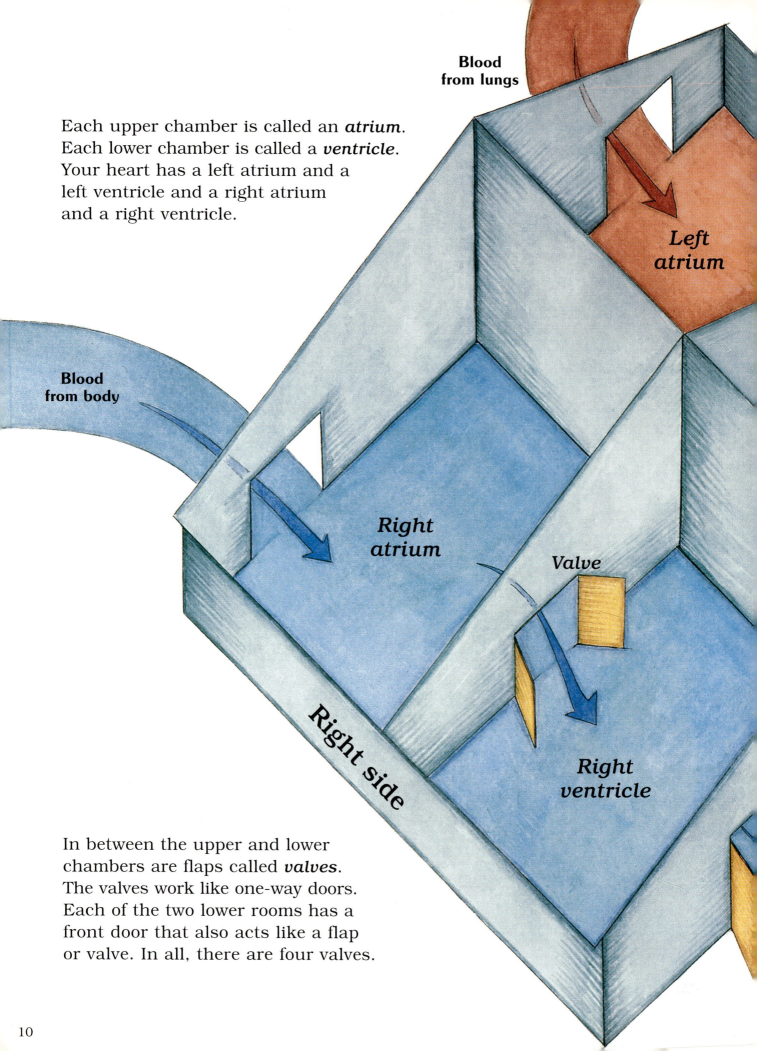

Each upper chamber is called an *atrium*. Each lower chamber is called a *ventricle*. Your heart has a left atrium and a left ventricle and a right atrium and a right ventricle.

Blood from lungs

Blood from body

Left atrium

Right atrium

Valve

Right side

Right ventricle

In between the upper and lower chambers are flaps called *valves*. The valves work like one-way doors. Each of the two lower rooms has a front door that also acts like a flap or valve. In all, there are four valves.

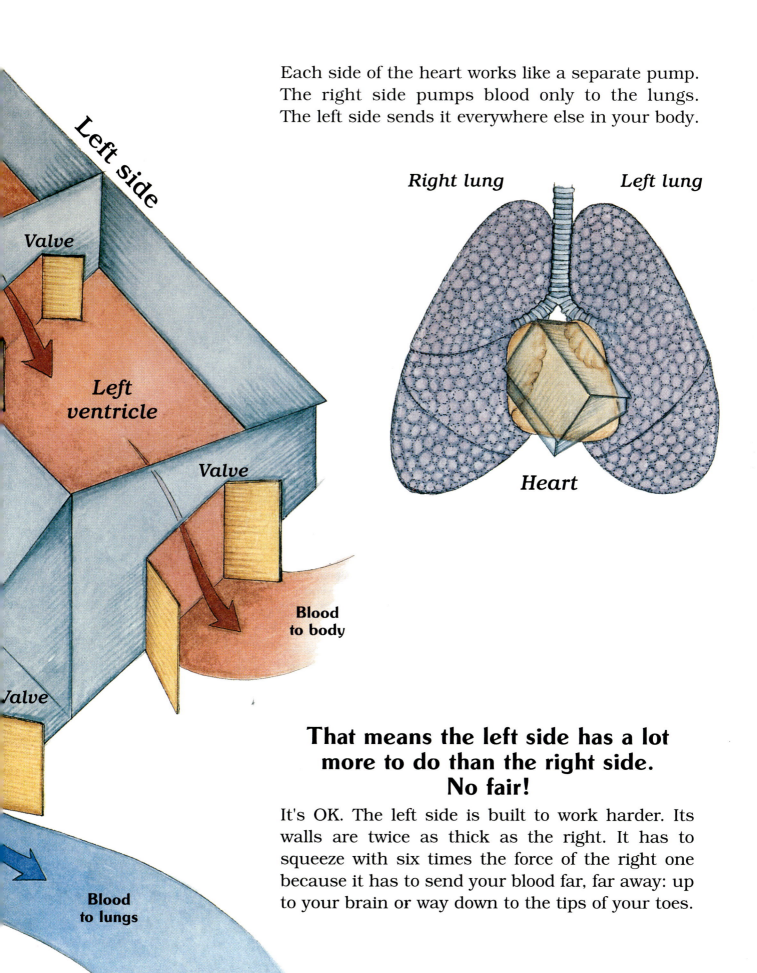

Left side

Valve

Left ventricle

Valve

Blood to body

Valve

Blood to lungs

Each side of the heart works like a separate pump. The right side pumps blood only to the lungs. The left side sends it everywhere else in your body.

Right lung   *Left lung*

Heart

That means the left side has a lot more to do than the right side. No fair!

It's OK. The left side is built to work harder. Its walls are twice as thick as the right. It has to squeeze with six times the force of the right one because it has to send your blood far, far away: up to your brain or way down to the tips of your toes.

Here's what happens.

The *tricuspid valve* opens so that blood flows through it from the right atrium to the right ventricle. Then electricity makes your heart squeeze, or *contract*.

SLAM!

The valve snaps shut.

Blood is pushed forward through the *pulmonic valve* to a big tube called the *pulmonary artery*. That will take it to the lungs.

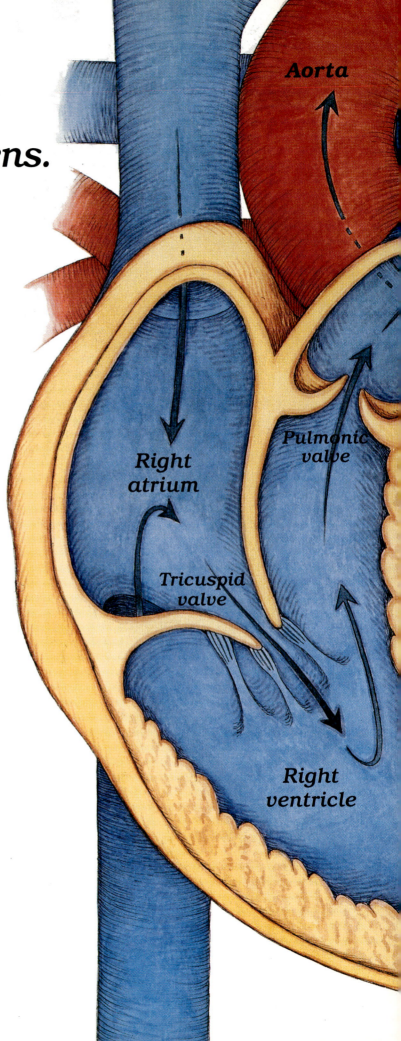

Aorta

Pulmonic valve

Right atrium

Tricuspid valve

Right ventricle

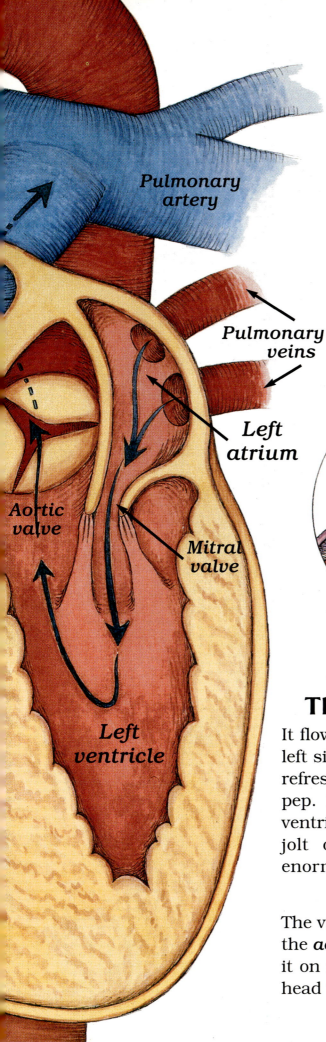

Pulmonary artery

Pulmonary veins

Left atrium

Aortic valve

Mitral valve

Left ventricle

Why does blood need to go to the lungs?

The blood in the right side of the heart contains wastes, including a waste gas called **carbon dioxide**. It needs oxygen. Luckily, there's plenty of that in the air. You bring oxygen in every time you take in a breath. So the blood picks up oxygen in your lungs and leaves behind carbon dioxide.

Where does the carbon dioxide go?

Out, thanks to you! You get rid of it every time you breathe out.

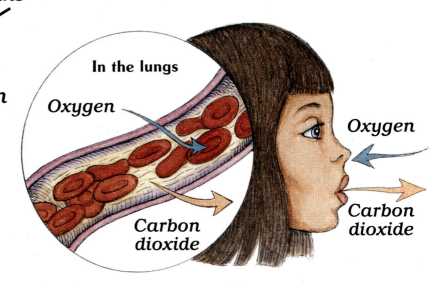

In the lungs

Oxygen

Oxygen

Carbon dioxide

Carbon dioxide

Then what happens to the blood?

It flows into the **pulmonary veins** and back to the left side of the heart. But it's changed because it's refreshed with oxygen. It's bright red and full of pep. It flows from the left atrium into the left ventricle through the **mitral valve**. Then the same jolt of your homemade electricity makes an enormous, tremendous squeeze.

SLAM!

The valve snaps shut and blood is pushed through the **aortic valve** into the **aorta**. The aorta will send it on its way through your whole body, from your head to your toes.

How can the aorta stretch through my whole body?

It doesn't. The aorta branches off into tubes that get smaller and smaller. It's as if you have roads of blood running through you. Some roads are wide, wide highways and some are narrow little alleys, but they're all connected.

Heads up

Blood is under such pressure when it leaves the left side of your heart that if the aorta were cut, blood would spurt out higher than your head.

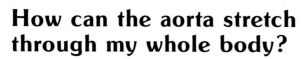

To Arm and Head

A

Valve from Heart

To a Leg

To a Leg

Keep on pumping

How much blood does our heart pump every day? Only a few ounces per beat. But since it beats so many times during 24 hours, it adds up to 1,250 gallons of blood pumped a day.

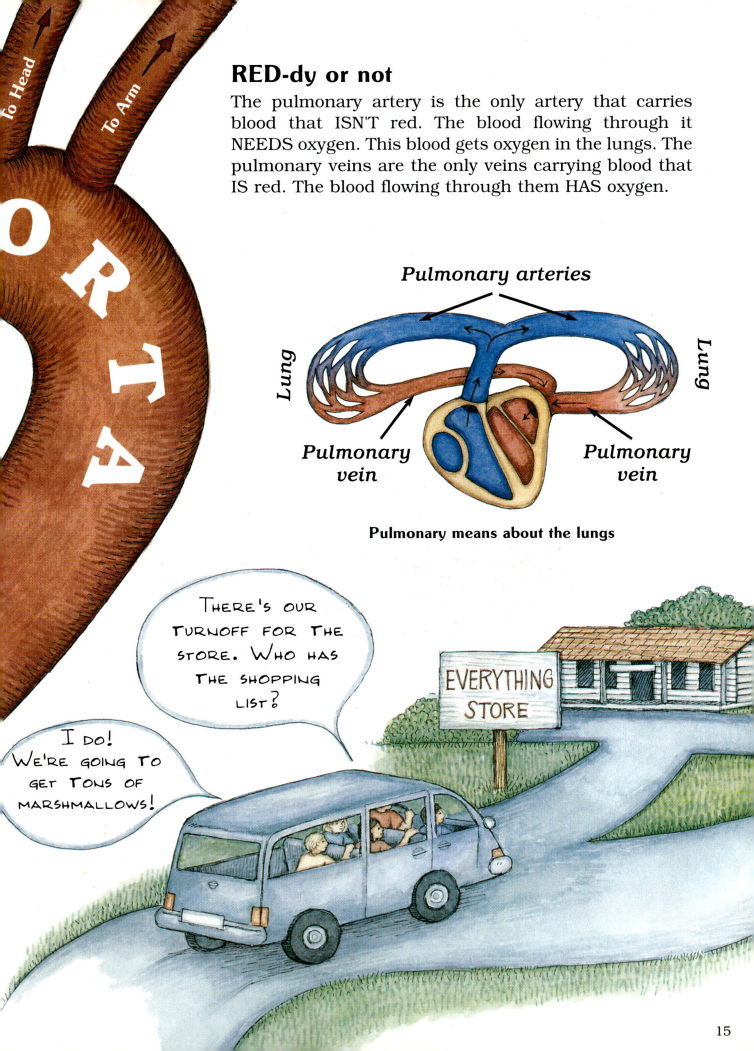

RED-dy or not

The pulmonary artery is the only artery that carries blood that ISN'T red. The blood flowing through it NEEDS oxygen. This blood gets oxygen in the lungs. The pulmonary veins are the only veins carrying blood that IS red. The blood flowing through them HAS oxygen.

Pulmonary arteries

Lung

Lung

Pulmonary vein

Pulmonary vein

Pulmonary means about the lungs

To Head

To Arm

ORTA

THERE'S OUR TURNOFF FOR THE STORE. WHO HAS THE SHOPPING LIST?

I DO! WE'RE GOING TO GET TONS OF MARSHMALLOWS!

EVERYTHING STORE

Round & Round It Goes . . .

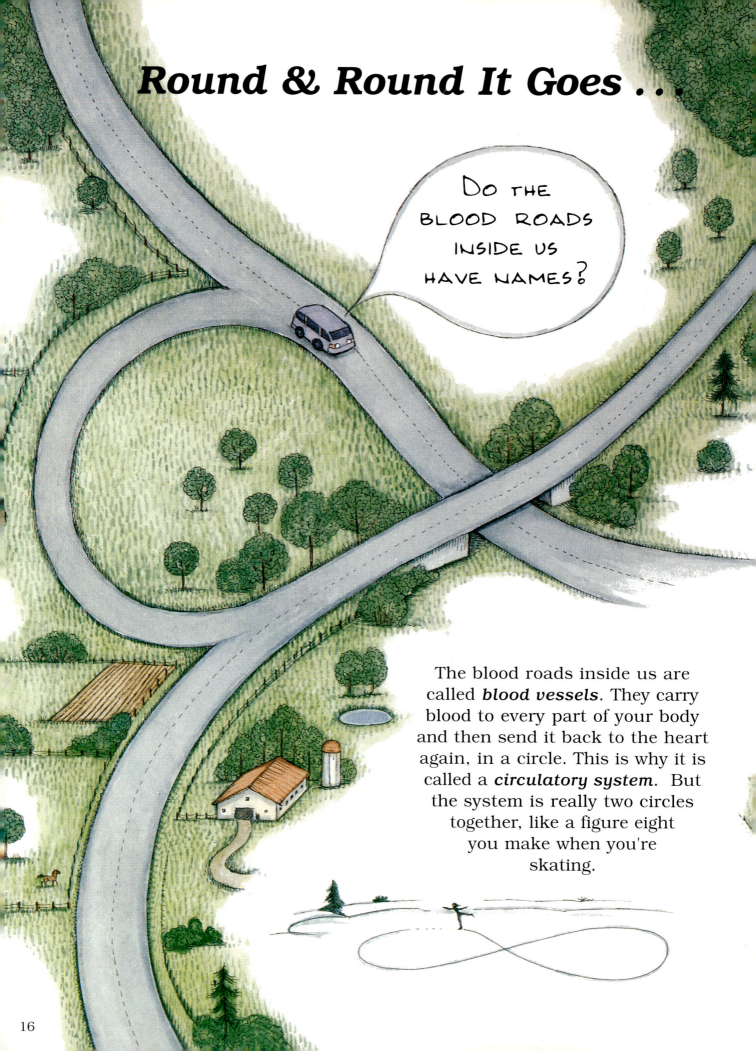

Do the blood roads inside us have names?

The blood roads inside us are called *blood vessels*. They carry blood to every part of your body and then send it back to the heart again, in a circle. This is why it is called a *circulatory system*. But the system is really two circles together, like a figure eight you make when you're skating.

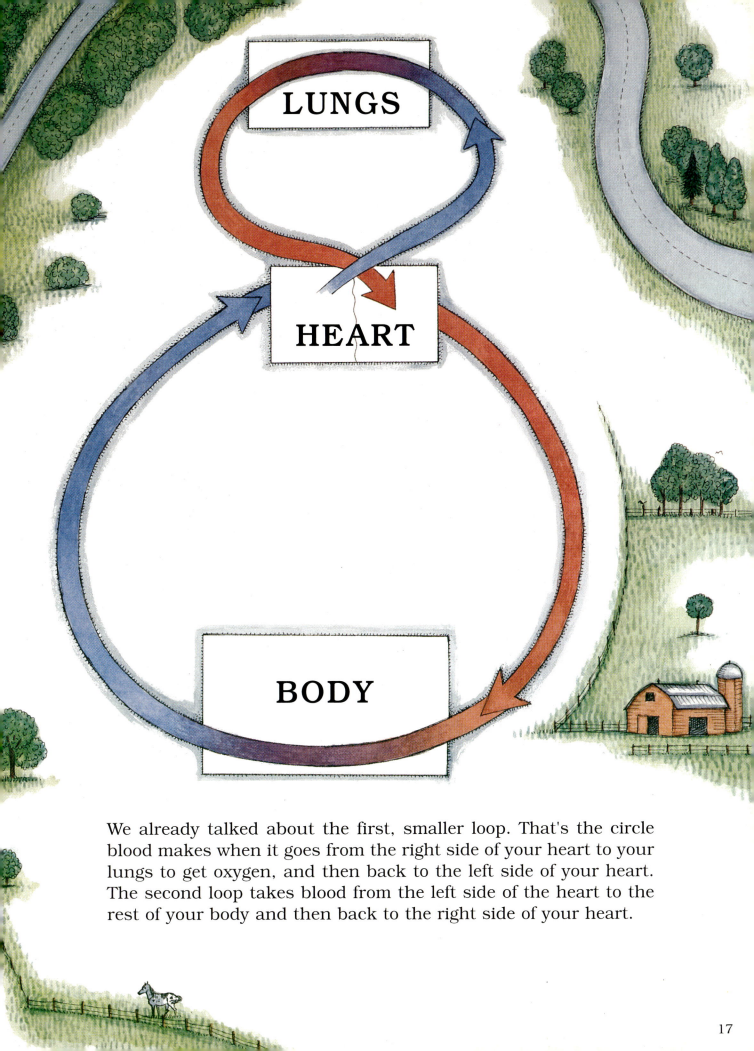

LUNGS

HEART

BODY

We already talked about the first, smaller loop. That's the circle blood makes when it goes from the right side of your heart to your lungs to get oxygen, and then back to the left side of your heart. The second loop takes blood from the left side of the heart to the rest of your body and then back to the right side of your heart.

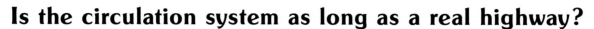

Is the circulation system as long as a real highway?

It's much, much longer than any road system in the world! If you could pull the blood vessels out of your body and lay them down end to end, they would stretch about 60,000 miles. That's more than twice around the world. You would have to walk for two years, fast, without ever once stopping, to reach the end.

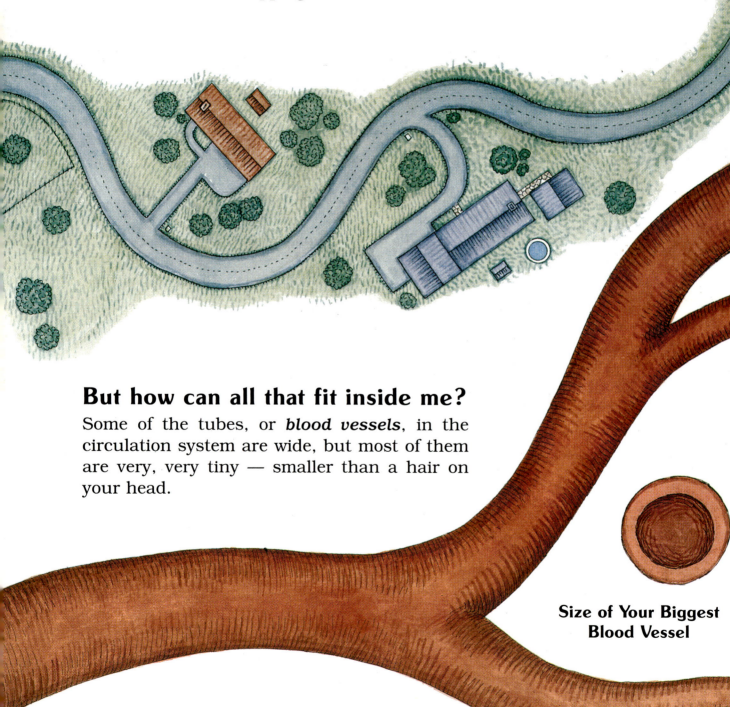

But how can all that fit inside me?

Some of the tubes, or *blood vessels*, in the circulation system are wide, but most of them are very, very tiny — smaller than a hair on your head.

Size of Your Biggest Blood Vessel

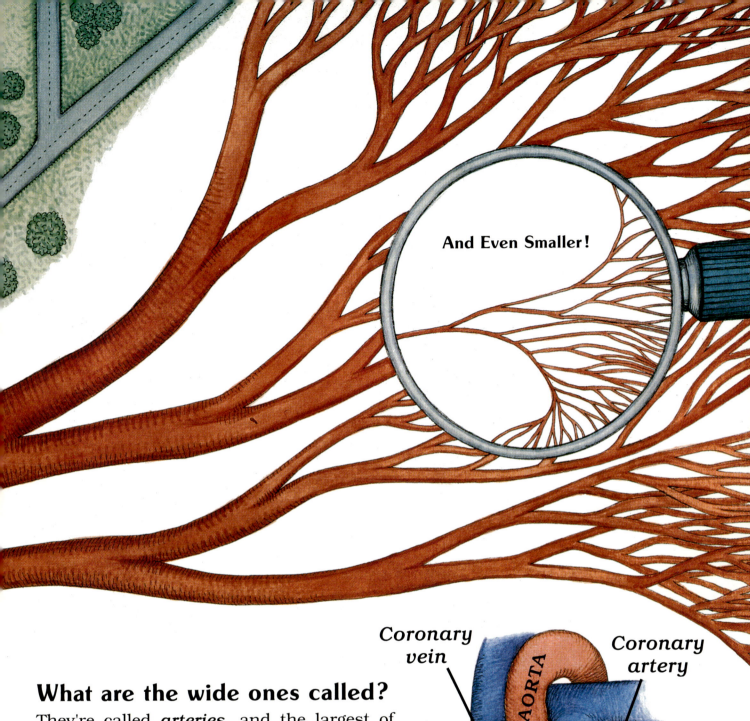

And Even Smaller!

What are the wide ones called?

They're called *arteries*, and the largest of them is your *aorta*. Blood rushes through the aorta to other arteries to feed your brain, liver, kidneys, and other body parts with oxygen and nutrients. Even your heart muscle gets fed. The *coronary arteries* carry blood to the heart muscle itself.

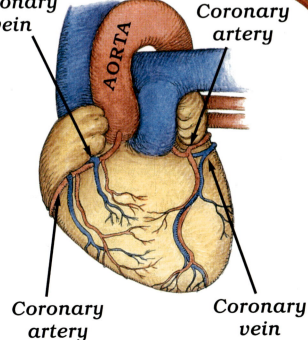

Coronary vein

Coronary artery

AORTA

Coronary artery

Coronary vein

"Coronary" means about the heart

Where does the blood go after it leaves the arteries?

Inside your organs, blood enters narrower tubes called *arterioles*, or little arteries. Then it squeezes into tiny vessels called *capillaries*. You have trillions and trillions of them. They're so narrow that blood cells have to line up single file to fit inside. While blood is in a capillary, oxygen, and other nutrients pass through its thin walls into cells. That's where the real feeding takes place. Then the blood picks up wastes such as carbon dioxide. It also picks up the good substances produced by the organs of the body.

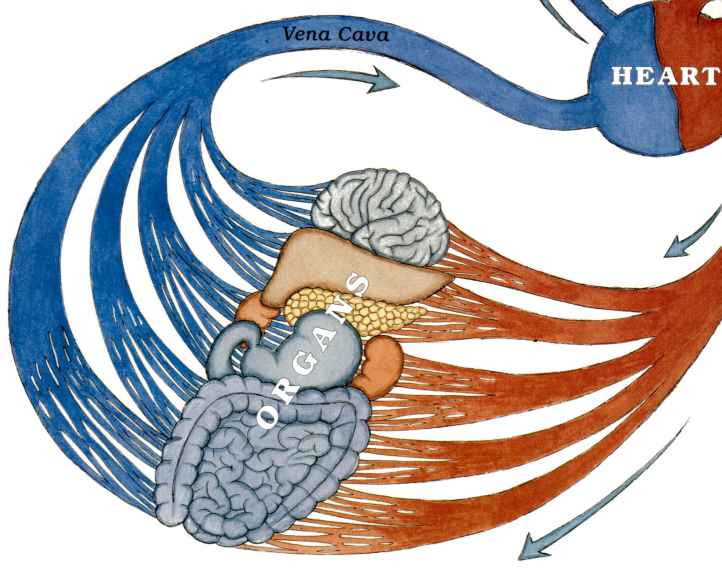

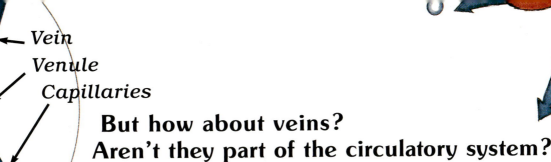

Vein
Venule
Capillaries

But how about veins?
Aren't they part of the circulatory system?

Veins are part of blood's return trip to the heart, after it's fed the organs. Blood flows from capillaries into little veins called *venules*. Those lead to bigger veins . . . then bigger . . . and then the biggest ones, the *vena cava*, which lead to the right side of the heart.

I'm getting tired just thinking about it.

So is your blood, by this time! It's lost oxygen and picked up waste and a lot of good substances. It then returns to the lungs for more oxygen and gives up carbon dioxide.

Oxygen

How long does that take? All day?

No. It all happens in less than *one minute*. Blood moves fast and smoothly when blood vessels are healthy and in good shape. But when they're not, there can be big trouble.

Don't be blue.

Why are veins blue? Because the blood in the veins has given up its reddening oxygen to your cells.

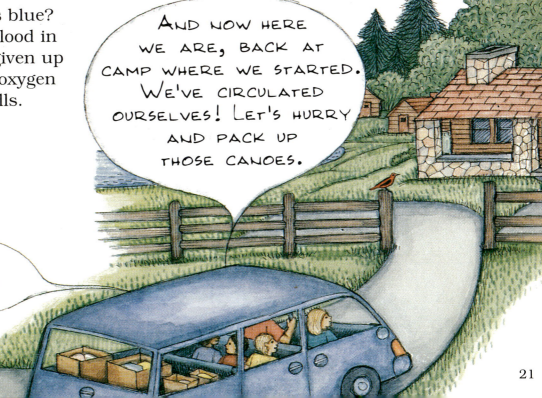

AND NOW HERE WE ARE, BACK AT CAMP WHERE WE STARTED. WE'VE CIRCULATED OURSELVES! LET'S HURRY AND PACK UP THOSE CANOES.

YAY!

21

Healthy Heart, Happy Heart

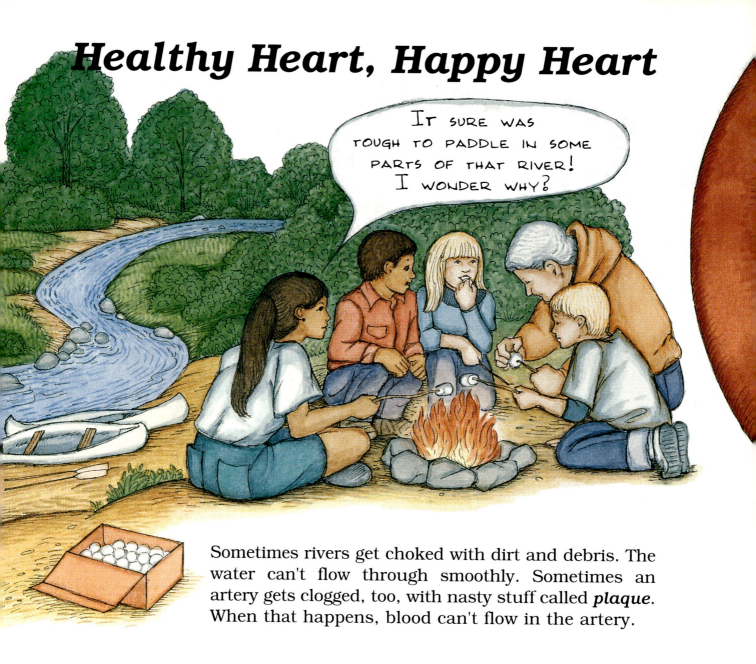

It sure was tough to paddle in some parts of that river! I wonder why?

Sometimes rivers get choked with dirt and debris. The water can't flow through smoothly. Sometimes an artery gets clogged, too, with nasty stuff called *plaque*. When that happens, blood can't flow in the artery.

What is plaque made of?

Plaque is made mainly of fat and a chemical called *cholesterol*. It can build up in arteries from the time we are teenagers. It isn't caused by one thing, but many things acting together. You can't change some of these things. For instance, some people make more plaque than others. But you *can* change some things.

Like what?

Like watching what you eat. If you cut down on foods with a lot of fat or cholesterol, you may reduce how much plaque your body makes. And smoking plays a big part in causing plaque. That's one reason you must NEVER smoke!

Can plaque make a person sick?

That depends on where the plaque is. If it builds up in the coronary arteries, it can block the blood flow to the heart muscle. This is the cause of the most common type of heart disease. Without enough blood to feed it, the heart muscle may hurt when you exercise. We call that type of pain *angina pectoris*. When the plaque sort of explodes abruptly, it may completely block the flow of blood in a coronary artery. When that happens, the heart muscle becomes damaged and has to work harder and harder to pump enough blood to your other organs. That's what happens during a *heart attack*.

Can kids have heart attacks?

Kids should not worry about getting heart attacks from plaque. It takes many years for plaque to build up in the arteries. But kids can do things right now to prevent plaque later. You can limit foods such as beef and pork and foods that are high in fat and cholesterol. Instead, you can eat a lot of vegetables and fruit and drink plenty of water and juice. You need to get plenty of exercise, too. Your heart is a muscle and it needs exercise like all your other muscles.

Do all kids have healthy hearts?

Sometimes babies are born with hearts whose valves, or some other part of the heart, is not quite right. But doctors usually notice those problems right away, and they can treat nearly all of them.

Plaque

Open Blood Vessel

How do I know my own heart's OK?

Just ask your doctor!

How do I know how much fat or cholesterol is in my food?

The amount of fat and cholesterol in most packaged foods is printed on the wrapper. Foods with a lot of fat and cholesterol include butter, whole milk, eggs, beef, bacon, ice cream, potato chips, and many kinds of cheese. Ask a teacher or other grown-up if you need help in understanding the information on food wrappers.

23

A few weeks later in the doctor's library

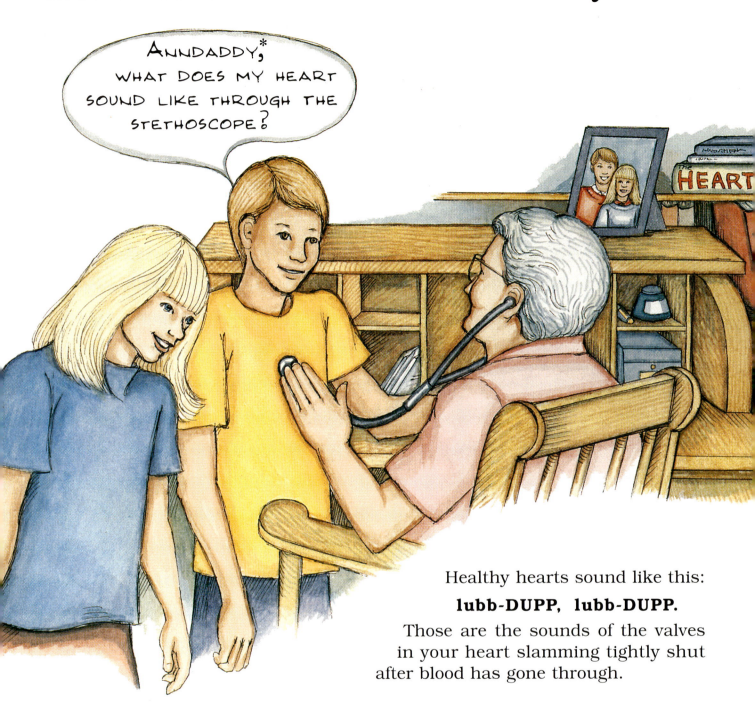

ANNDADDY,* WHAT DOES MY HEART SOUND LIKE THROUGH THE STETHOSCOPE?

Healthy hearts sound like this:

lubb-DUPP, lubb-DUPP.

Those are the sounds of the valves in your heart slamming tightly shut after blood has gone through.

What does a sick heart sound like?

It would depend on the problem. A very loud **lupp** might mean the mitral valve isn't working right. A soft **DUPP** could mean the aortic valve is in trouble. Or a new noise called a *murmur* could be heard. It might sound like a bowling ball rolling down an alley or like someone clearing his throat. A doctor can recognize these sounds and determine what they mean.

* *Look this up in the Preface of this book.*

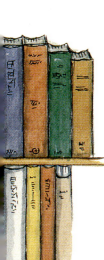

How fast does my heart beat?

The younger you are, the faster it goes. Babies' hearts can beat 130 times a minute. Grown-up hearts beat 70 or 75 times a minute. Yours is somewhere in between: about 85 times a minute.

Why does this cuff feel so tight?

I'm taking your blood pressure. The cuff squeezes the muscles in your upper arm so no blood goes through — but not long enough to hurt you, so don't worry! With the cuff squeezed tight, I don't hear anything through my stethoscope. But when I start to loosen the cuff, the blood starts moving and I can hear some sounds. The machine attached to the cuff turns those sounds into two numbers, one for your heart at work, when it beats, and one when it's at rest between beats. Blood pressure that is higher than normal must be treated because it can damage the heart, kidneys, and brain. It also contributes to plaque.

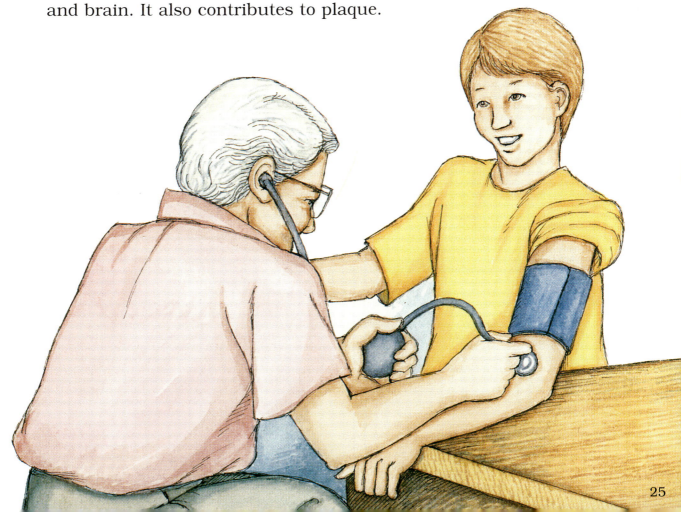

What if we want to know more about how our hearts are working?

First I would ask if you had certain feelings called *symptoms* like pains in your chest or feeling out of breath. Next I would take your pulse and blood pressure, look at the veins in your neck, and listen to your heart sounds. An x-ray film of your chest could tell me even more about your heart. And there's a special machine, called an electrocardiograph, that can tell me if your heart is making normal or abnormal waves of electricity.

Doctors have lots of ways to tell how your heart is working. But we can't do the most important thing: stop disease from harming your heart in the first place. *That's up to you.*

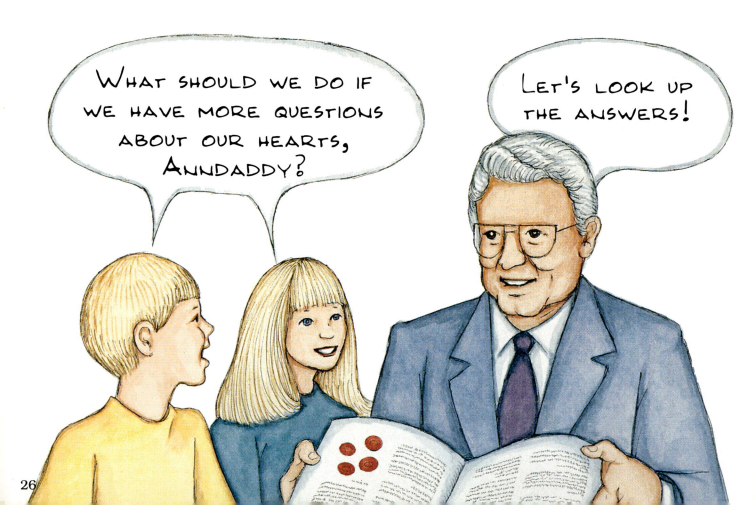

How can I do that?

You must exercise and eat less fat and more vegetables and fruit. In addition, it's up to you to have your blood pressure checked and treated if it's too high. And you must stay away from three really bad guys: bad drugs, smoking, and alcohol. Each one is out to get your heart in its own terrible way. Smoking can narrow arteries and make clots. It can also cause lung diseases that will leave you gasping for breath or dragging around an oxygen tank for air. Drinking alcohol can also damage your heart muscle.

There's no doubt about it: Your heart needs YOU to keep it safe from these heart-hurters! We doctors can help with some of the new and wonderful drugs and surgery, but you and you alone can help *prevent* plaque in the coronary and other arteries.

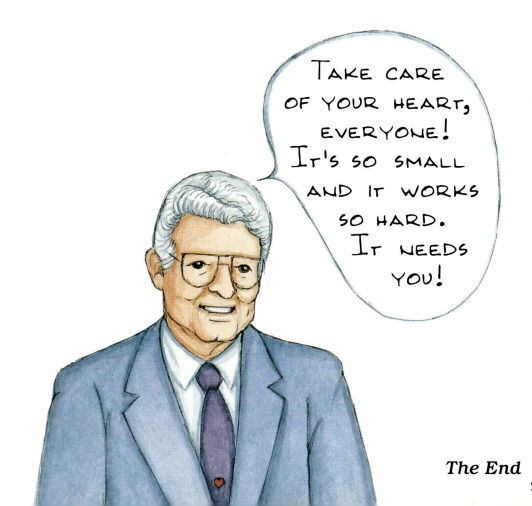

TAKE CARE OF YOUR HEART, EVERYONE! IT'S SO SMALL AND IT WORKS SO HARD. IT NEEDS YOU!

The End

Glossary

Aorta (ay-OR-tuh)
The largest artery in your body. The aorta carries blood from your heart to the rest of your body.

Arteries
Blood vessels branching off the aorta. Arteries carry blood away from the heart.

Arterioles
Smaller blood vessels branching off arteries.

Atrium (AY-tree-um)
One of the two upper chambers of the heart. Your heart has a right atrium and a left atrium.

Capillaries
The smallest blood vessels. Inside your organs, capillaries exchange nutrients and oxygen for carbon dioxide, and good and bad substances made by the organs.

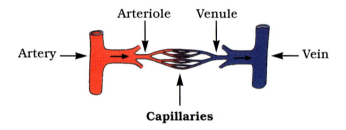

Capillaries

Cells
The tiny "building blocks" that make up part of every living thing. You need a microscope to see cells.

Cholesterol
A fatty chemical found in many foods. Foods high in cholesterol can be dangerous to your heart.

Circulatory system
The flow of blood from the heart through the blood vessels around the body and back to the heart.

Congenital (kun-JEN-i-tul) heart disease
Problems or defects of the heart that people are born with.

Coronary (CORE-uh-nair-ee) arteries
The arteries that carry blood to the heart muscle. Coronary arteries are called that because they "crown" the heart.

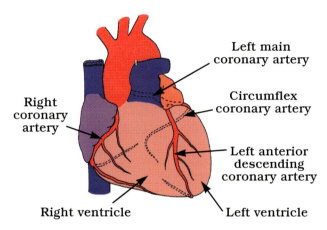

Coronary Arteries

Coronary atherosclerosis (a-thur-oh-sklur-OH-sis)
A kind of heart disease caused by fatty deposits that block the flow of blood in the coronary arteries.

Diastole (di-as-to-le)
When the heart relaxes. The mitral and tricuspid valves open. The aortic and pulmonary valves are closed.

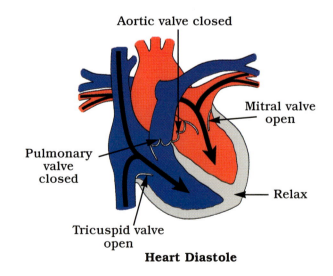

Heart Diastole

Electrical system
Electricity is made in the sinus node. It spreads to the AV node, His bundle, and bundle branches.

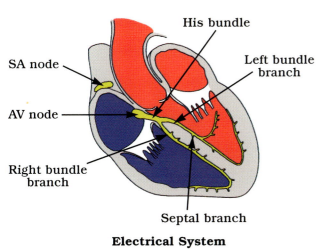

Electrical System

Electrocardiogram
A graph showing the electrical waves made in your heart.

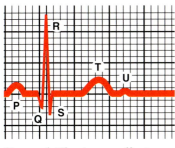

Normal Electrocardiogram

Endothelium (en-do-thel-i-um)
Cells that make the inner lining of the arteries and veins. These cells make a lot of active chemicals.

Heart attack
A serious medical condition that happens when the blood flow in a coronary artery is suddenly blocked.

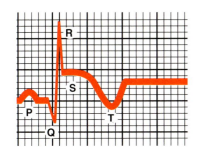

Electrocardiogram of Heart Attack

Heart disease
Disease of the heart valves, coronary arteries, the heart muscle tissue itself, or the electrical system of the heart.

Heart
The muscular organ that pumps blood around your body.

Lungs
A pair of organs in your chest that bring in oxygen and let out carbon dioxide.

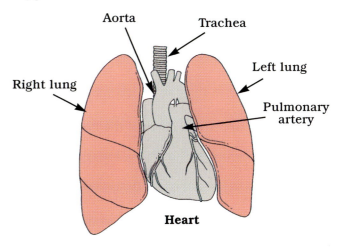

Heart

Murmur
A noise heard through a stethoscope that means a heart valve is either leaking blood or blocking the flow of blood.

Myocardium (my-oh-car-dee-um)
The heart muscle.

Oxygen
The life-giving gas that works with food and other nutrients, supplies energy to the cells of the body.

Plaque
A fatty substance that collects in the arteries. When it blocks the flow of blood in the coronary arteries it causes heart disease. Plaque can build up in other arteries and cause other serious medical conditions.

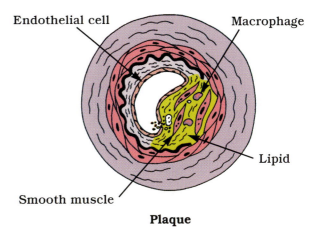

Plaque

Pulmonary (PULL-moh-nair-ee) artery
The artery that leads from your heart to your lungs. It's the only artery carrying blood that is NOT red.

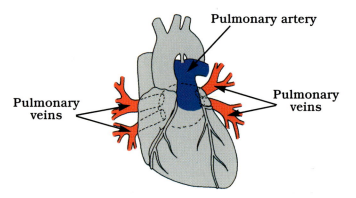

Pulmonary artery

Pulmonary veins

Pulmonary veins

Pulmonary Artery and Veins

Pulmonary veins
The veins that lead from your lungs to your heart. They're the only veins carrying blood that IS red.

Sphygmomanometer (sfig-mom-uh-NAH-muh-ter)
A machine doctors use to measure blood pressure.

Stethoscope
An instrument with a small cup at one end that doctors use to listen to sounds inside your body, especially your heart and lungs.

Systole (sis-to-le)
When the heart squeezes. The aortic and pulmonary valves open. The tricuspid and mitral valves close.

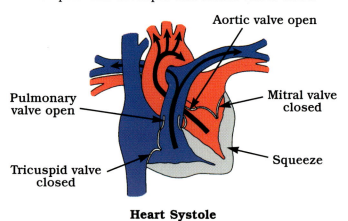

Aortic valve open

Pulmonary valve open

Mitral valve closed

Tricuspid valve closed

Squeeze

Heart Systole

Valves
Flaps in your heart and veins that work like one-way doors, preventing blood from flowing backwards.

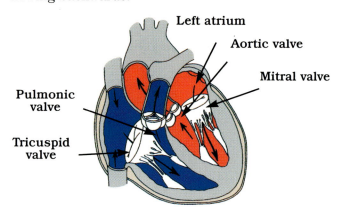

Left atrium

Aortic valve

Mitral valve

Pulmonic valve

Tricuspid valve

Valves of the Heart

Veins
Blood vessels that carry blood toward the heart.

Vena cava (VEE-nuh CAVE-uh)
The body's largest vein, which carries blood to the right side of your heart. There are actually two: the *inferior vena cava*, which carries blood from the lower part of your body and the *superior vena cava*, which carries blood from the upper part.

Ventricle
One of the two lower chambers of the heart. Your heart has a right ventricle and a left ventricle.

Venules (VEH-nyoolz)
Smaller blood vessels branching out from veins.

References

Carnegie Library, Science & Technology Departments. *Handy Science Answer Book*. Pittsburgh: Visible Ink Press (Gale Research), 1994.

Hurst, J.W. (editor-in-chief), R. C. Schlant (assoc. ed.), and C. E. Rackley, E. H. Sonnenblick, and N. K. Wenger (eds.). *The Heart: Arteries and Veins*. 7th ed. New York: McGraw-Hill, 1990.

Weekly Reader Books. *Young Students Learning Library*. Funk & Wagnalls and Field Publications, 1988. p. 551.